PURE HONOKIOL
ONE EXTRACT, MANY BENEFITS

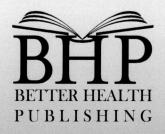

BHP
BETTER HEALTH
PUBLISHING

The purpose of this book is to educate. It is not intended to serve as a replacement for professional medical advice. Any use of the information in this book is at the reader's discretion. This book is sold with the understanding that neither the publisher nor the author has any liability or responsibility for any injury caused or alleged to be caused directly or indirectly by the information in this book. While every effort has been made to ensure its accuracy, the book's contents should not be construed as medical advice.

To obtain medical advice on your individual health needs, please consult a qualified health care practitioner.

First Edition Copyright ©2013 Better Health Publishing

All rights reserved. No part of this publication may be reproduced, stored in a retrieval system, or transmitted in any form or any means, electronic, mechanical, photocopying, recording, or otherwise, without the prior written permission of the publisher.

Published by Better Health Publishing, Santa Rosa, CA

Printed in the United States of America

Contents

Foreword by Dr. Isaac Eliaz i
1. The Cutting Edge of Cancer Care 1
2. Attacking Cancer from all Sides 5
3. Synergy with Cancer Treatments 10
4. Inflammation and Oxidation 13
5. Neural Protection 15
6. Healthy Mood Support 17
7. Cardiovascular, Metabolic, Immune Health and more... 20
8. The Future of Honokiol 24
Appendix 1. How to Use Honokiol 26
Appendix ii. References & Research 28
Appendix iii. Index 34

Foreword by Dr. Isaac Eliaz

"It's rare to find one therapeutic agent that delivers so many benefits against cancer and chronic disease."

Advancements in herbal extraction methods and innovations in nutritional sciences have greatly expanded our pharmacopeia of powerful, natural medicines. As an integrative cancer physician and researcher, I actively seek out important new botanical compounds and nutrients that can be combined into a comprehensive program to fight cancer and restore health. A key strategy in integrative oncology is to apply multiple treatments which exert different mechanisms of action, in order to fight cancer from multiple angles.

It's rare to find one therapeutic agent that delivers so many benefits against cancer and chronic disease. Honokiol is one of these unique and remarkable compounds. There are now hundreds of peer-reviewed studies demonstrating the extensive actions of this botanical extract, particularly in the treatment and prevention of aggressive cancer.

Honokiol is an active ingredient derived from the bark of the *Magnolia officinalis* tree. For thousands of years, traditional Chinese herbalists and doctors relied on Magnolia bark to treat a wide range of illnesses. Today, advanced extraction methods have succeeded in isolating and purifying the active ingredient Honokiol from raw magnolia bark. The result is that we've discovered a remarkable new therapy to add to our growing repertoire of safe and effective, powerful natural medicines.

The Search

Compelled by the research and reports from fellow clinicians, I began my search for the highest quality Honokiol. A handful of my cancer patients had also studied Honokiol's fast-growing body of published literature, and were interested in using it with other therapies. One of Honokiol's most impressive anti-cancer effects can be found in its ability to boost conventional cancer treatments like radiation and chemotherapy — even re-sensitizing the cancer to drugs that had previously failed.

After extensive analysis and rigorous testing, my team of researchers and I sourced the highest quality, 98% purified Honokiol extract for clinical use. The results have been nothing short of remarkable. Clinical observations continue to substantiate the published research on this powerful ingredient, showing Honokiol to be one of the most important natural anti-cancer agents with a wide range of additional applications.

Extensive Benefits

In published research, Honokiol demonstrates an astonishing array of therapeutic actions:

- Anti-tumor
- Anti-metastasis
- Antioxidant
- Selective pro-oxidant against cancer
- Anti-inflammatory
- Antibacterial
- Glucose balance
- Cardiovascular support
- Neural and cognitive sup
- Immune support
- Anti-anxiety
- Antidepressant
- Other actions and benefi

Forward by Dr. Isaac Eliaz | iii

Furthermore, pure Honokiol is safe and effective, absorbs quickly and works synergistically with many botanicals, supplements and conventional treatments. With such a diverse array of powerful effects, Honokiol has become a critical component in strategic, integrative health protocols. Within a targeted anti-cancer program, Honokiol may offer the critical advantage needed to overcome this all-too-common disease.

While there are no magic bullets against any chronic disease, Honokiol stands out as an incredibly versatile and powerful natural healer with an essential role in integrative cancer care.

If you have concerns about cancer or other chronic health issues, I encourage you to read this guide, and share it with anyone you know who wants to learn more about the remarkable benefits of this unique ingredient.

In best health,

Isaac Eliaz, M.D., M.S., L.Ac.

Medical Director,
Amitabha Medical Clinic

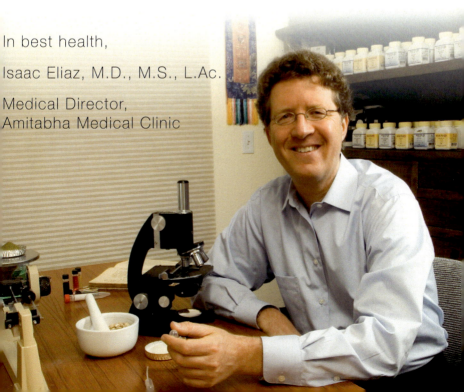

The Cutting Edge of Cancer Care

Successful integrative cancer treatments are built on a dynamic, multidimensional strategy to increase overall health while fighting the disease. Honokiol's ability to block the growth and spread of cancer on the cellular and genomic levels, combined with its powerful antioxidant and anti-inflammatory properties, make it a highly strategic component within integrative cancer treatments.

Equally important, Honokiol shows the ability to reverse chemotherapy resistance and allow certain chemotherapy drugs to work more effectively, which we'll explore later in this book. This can mean the difference between life and death for patients who have been failed by existing therapies. Honokiol is also shown to improve radiation treatment and help reduce painful side effects. Honokiol's powerful synergistic abilities are a key reason why it plays such an important role within integrative cancer protocols.

In fact, Honokiol offers both preventive and active therapeutic benefits. On the preventive side, Honokiol helps reduce the cancer-promoting oxidation and inflammation caused by free radicals, toxins and heavy metals. Over-oxidation is particularly worrisome, as it can damage DNA, promoting abnormal cell growth and cancer development. Honokiol also boosts immunity and supports circulation, two key components of cancer prevention and control.

Crossing the Blood-Brain Barrier

The blood-brain barrier is critical to neural health. It restricts the size of particles entering the brain, protecting us from bacterial infections and other conditions. Unfortunately, that protection also keeps out beneficial therapies, such as chemotherapeutic agents, making it more difficult to treat brain cancer.

Honokiol is a very small molecule, so it can easily enter the circulation and travel throughout the body to reach targeted areas quickly. This small molecular size also allows it to cross the blood-brain barrier, where Honokiol has been proven helpful against brain cancer and other neurological diseases. In particular, a 2011 study published in *PLoS One* showed that Honokiol crossed the blood-brain barrier and inhibited gliosarcoma (brain) tumors in animals. Gliosarcomas are among the most difficult cancers to treat.

Multiple Anti-Cancer Functions

On the cellular level, Honokiol actively blocks a number of specific cancer mechanisms. Remember, cancer is a disease of uncontrolled cellular growth, and rapid growth requires increased nutrition. One of cancer's survival tactics is to create new blood vessel supplies to the tumor, a process called angiogenesis. More blood vessels mean more food for the tumor and faster growth and metastasis to other organs.

Researched in Multiple Cancers

Extensive research has shown that Honokiol:

- Boosts apoptosis in pancreatic cancer cells
- Inhibits prostate cancer cells
- Prevents breast cancer cells from growing and metastasizing
- Stops brain tumor growth
- Boosts apoptosis in oral cancer cells
- Induces rapid cancer cell death in metastatic bone cancer
- Inhibits non-small cell lung cancer cells
- Inhibits gastric cancer cells
- Inhibits adult T cell leukemia
- Inhibits colon cancer cells
- Inhibits malignant melanoma and prevents other skin cancers
- Works with other treatments to increase their anti-cancer activity
- Suppresses numerous pro-cancer genes and proteins
- Offers numerous primary *and* secondary anti-cancer benefits

onokiol works in part to halt angiogenesis, thus helping prevent tumor growth and metastasis. For example, a 012 study published in *PLoS One* showed Honokiol's ility to block angiogenesis and proliferation of gastric ancer cells by regulating specific cell signaling athways.

ut cancer is also a disease of failed quality control, to speak. Normally, unhealthy, mutated or abnormal cells have a quality control checkpoint that causes the diseased cells to self-destruct and die. This is an important regulatory process called apoptosis. However, cancer disables apoptosis, allowing tumor cells to grow and even survive chemotherapy, radiation and other treatments.

By disabling angiogenesis and boosting apoptosis in cancer cells throughout the body, Honokiol provides a powerful one-two punch against tumor growth and metastasis. But it also shows the ability to kill cancer cells directly, unrelated to apoptosis and cellular quality control.

For example, a 2012 study in the journal *Cancer* explored Honokiol's ability to cause rapid cell death in metastatic bone cancer. Researchers observed that this specific anti-cancer mechanism did not involve self-destruction/apoptosis of cancer cells. Instead, higher concentrations of Honokiol attacked and killed aggressive bone cancer cells *directly*. Such powerful, direct cytotoxic activity against cancer cells gives Honokiol yet another unique advantage in the fight against this deadly disease.

In the next chapter, we'll take a closer look at what scientists have discovered about Honokiol's remarkable anti-cancer effects at the cellular and genetic levels.

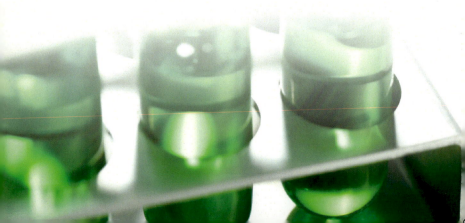

Attacking Cancer from all Sides

In some ways, cancer is like an under-filled water balloon: It's difficult to pop it with one hand, because no matter how hard you squeeze, parts of the balloon keep poking through your fingers. Even two hands may not cover all the escape routes. Similarly, a single cancer treatment may kill 98 percent of the disease; however, the remaining two percent may be resistant to treatment, allowing the tumor to return.

Because cancer is such a complex and rapidly changing disease, dynamic therapies must be combined to attack it from multiple angles. A primary goal is staying ahead of the disease to prevent it from evading treatment. Therefore, one approach, no matter how strong, is rarely enough. Nevertheless, with such a wide range of therapeutic actions, Honokiol is one of the single most powerful natural anti-cancer agents. And as research continues, it may likely be considered one of the most important.

Honokiol excels as an anti-cancer strategy because it performs so many tasks so well. Cancer thrives on inflammation and oxidation. Honokiol acts swiftly against both, while inhibiting angiogenesis, fighting cancer growth and reducing proliferation. It also provides a wealth of additional benefits that will be explored throughout this book.

Lastly, Honokiol exerts its powerful effects safely without causing significant side effects—in fact it helps to reduce the severity of side effects triggered by conventional treatments.

Helps Malignant Cells Self-Destruct

Cellular signaling is a finely tuned system that ensures effective communication between cells and within cells. This is especially important for the cell cycle, the process through which cells grow and divide. For example, our DNA has 3 billion base pairs, each of which must be perfectly replicated when a cell divides. Errors can lead to mutations, which can cause cancer.

Cells do make mistakes, but sophisticated quality control systems inside the cell are supposed to catch and correct these problems. For example, cell cycle checkpoints stop DNA replication to ensure everything is going as planned. If not, and there's too much damage, the cell enters apoptosis, or programmed cell death. In other words, damaged cells are supposed to self-destruct. However, cancer cells find clever ways to disable this system and continue growing uncontrollably.

Honokiol actively influences cell communication, regulating DNA replication and stimulating apoptosis in cancerous and abnormal cells. In 2011, a study published in *PLoS One* found that Honokiol arrests the cell cycle and induces apoptosis in pancreatic cancer cells. The study also showed that Honokiol enhances the apoptotic effects of the anti-cancer drug Gemcitabine.

In the treatment of leukemia, Honokiol induced cell cycle arrest and apoptosis through the inhibition of specific cancer cell survival signals. This data was published in 2012 in the journal *Biochimica et Biophysica Acta*.

A 2012 study in the *American Journal of Surgery* showed Honokiol's ability to stop the proliferation and spread of malignant melanoma. Melanoma is one of the deadliest cancers because it grows and metastasizes so quickly. In this study, Honokiol induced cancer cell death and blocked proliferation by regulating cell cycle arrest through multiple signaling pathways.

Another study in the *International Journal of Oral Science* found that Honokiol induced apoptosis in oral squamous cell carcinoma.

In non-small cell lung cancer, which represents approximately 80% of lung cancer cases, Honokiol suppressed cancer cell growth and induced apoptosis. Results of this 2013 study were published in the journal *Epigenetics*, again showing Honokiol's anti-cancer effects through its influence on multiple cell signaling pathways. In this study, cell cycle checkpoints were re-activated leading to apoptosis and inhibition of specific pro-tumor proteins.

By reactivating critical cell cycle quality control mechanisms, Honokiol helps ensure that slightly damaged cells get fixed and thoroughly damaged cells, including malignant ones, die off.

Protects Precious Genomes

When error correction circuits go awry, mutations can occur that lead to cancer. What's worse, once cancer is in full effect, quality control mechanisms continue to unravel, leading to further mutations that can make tumors more aggressive, more treatment-resistant or both.

One quality control protein, called P53, suppresses tumors by preventing mutations. Cancer attacks this protein as part of its survival strategy. However, a 2009 review in the journal *Antioxidants & Redox Signaling*, gathered evidence showing that Honokiol blocks signals in tumors with defective P53 proteins. In addition, the study confirms Honokiol's ability to boost apoptosis in cancer cells.

Controls a Well Known Cancer Protein

Cancer often hijacks normal proteins to help it grow and survive. Like P53, NF-kB is important to the cell cycle, supporting normal growth; however, cancer mutates NF-kB so it never turns off. As a result, cells divide recklessly and resist apoptosis.

Excessive NF-kB activity can trigger cancer cell growth, invasion, proliferation and angiogenesis. Down-regulating the activity of NF-kB prevents cancer growth and metastasis, helps regulate the inflammation response and prevents cellular damage from oxidation. Honokiol suppresses overactive NF-kB, allowing the cell cycle to proceed normally.

Honokiol demonstrates remarkable synergy with numerous other ingredients, drugs, medicines and compounds, enhancing their beneficial effects. There are more than 800 therapeutic agents that inhibit NF-kB, including green tea and curcumin. Honokiol is shown to work with these agents, enhancing their impact for more powerful results. In the next chapter we'll take a closer look at how Honokiol works to improve other cancer treatments and strategies.

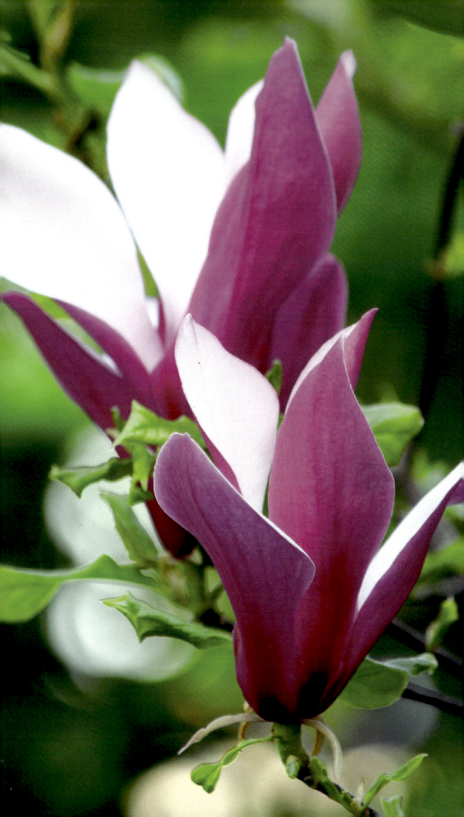

Synergy with Cancer Treatments

One of Honokiol's most impressive benefits is its ability to synergize with other cancer treatments. In other words, it can enhance the effectiveness of many different cancer fighting agents, both conventional and holistic. The whole becomes greater than the sum of its parts. Honokiol's unmatched synergistic effect delivers a critical advantage to any integrative anti-cancer program.

Overcomes Treatment Resistance

We recognize cancer by its rampant growth and spread throughout the body. But perhaps its most insidious trait is the ability to develop drug resistance. The initial happiness when a patient responds to treatment is often tempered as many cancers come roaring back. If we are going to cure cancer, we must solve the resistance problem.

Because cancer cells mutate so readily, they find ways to resist chemotherapy, radiotherapy, hormonal and natural treatments. Quite often, treatments that once destroyed tumors become ineffective. Even one mutation in a small group of cancer cells can make a big difference. That's why integrative cancer treatments are designed to stay one step ahead of the disease, and Honokiol may be one of the most powerful weapons in this strategy.

A number of studies have confirmed that Honokiol can decrease drug resistance in glioma, breast, prostate and other cancers. In fact, new investigations are helping us understand how Honokiol defeats cancer resistance.

Research in the *International Journal of Oncology* and other publications shows that Honokiol is adept at fighting treatment-resistant cancers by re-sensitizing cancer cells to chemotherapy and radiation treatments. As a result, a failed treatment is transformed into a successful one, providing new hope for many patients. Honokiol can even inhibit aggressive cancers that were previously considered untreatable.

One of the mechanisms cancer cells use to evade toxic treatments is to pump medicine out of the cell. Tiny protein pumps decrease cancer's sensitivity to treatments, allowing just enough cells to survive. These treatment-resistant cells grow rapidly to reconstitute the tumor.

However, a recent study showed that Honokiol can inhibit these pumps and restore cancer cell sensitivity to treatment. This is amazing news for cancer patients, many of whom will see their treatment options expand.

Further research highlights:

- A 2013 study published in the *International Journal of Oncology* showed that Honokiol synergized with chemotherapy drugs in multidrug resistant breast cancer.

- A 2012 study published in *Molecular Cancer Therapeutics* showed Honokiol resensitized treatment-resistant colon cancer stem cells to radiation therapy.

- A 2011 study in *PLoS One* found that Honokiol enhanced the apoptotic effects of the anti-cancer drug Gemcitabine against pancreatic cancer.

- Research published in *Oncology Letters* in 2011 found Honokiol enhanced the action of Cisplatin against colon cancer.

- A 2010 study from the *Journal of Biological Regulators Homeostatic Agents* showed that Honokiol resensitized cancer cells to Doxorubicin in multidrug resistant uterine cancer.

- A 2010 study in *Toxicology Mechanics Methodology* showed Honokiol performed synergistically with the drug Imatinib against human leukemia cells.

In addition to enhancing the therapeutic effects of chemotherapy and radiation, Honokiol shows powerful synergistic effects when combined with natural medicines, such as Modified Citrus Pectin (MCP). In one pre-published study, a combination of MCP and pure Honokiol dramatically decreased the proliferation of prostate cancer cells.

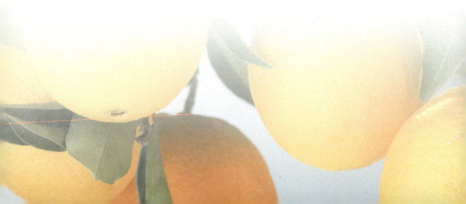

Inflammation and Oxidation

We have a strong incentive to support the body's ability to control oxidative stress. The damage caused by over-oxidation has been linked to cancer, heart disease, neurodegenerative diseases and other conditions.

When not modulated in some way, oxygen can be a destroying force—for example, consider how it reacts with iron and produces rust. However, oxidation is also a crucial biological process. Our immune system uses oxidation to destroy invaders. On the other hand, too much oxidation from unstable free radicals and reactive oxygen species (ROS) leads to inflammation and oxidative stress, interfering with normal processes and damaging proteins and DNA. While the body has a number of ways to reduce oxidation and fight free radicals, there are times when these processes just can't keep up.

Honokiol helps remove reactive oxygen from the body. In fact, as an antioxidant this compound demonstrates 1,000 times more free radical scavenging activity than Vitamin E. Studies have shown that Honokiol can help cells overcome oxidative stress, even extending into the nucleus to protect our DNA. Other research has found that Honokiol's anti-oxidative effects help prevent oxidized cholesterol and plaque buildup in blood vessels, protecting us from cardiovascular disease and stroke.

Controls Inflammation

Like oxidation, inflammation is a key part of the immune response. However, chronic inflammation can also lead to cancer, heart disease and other degenerative conditions. Obviously, fighting inflammation and reactive oxygen can have profound implications for good health. For example, one 2011 study in the journal *Intensive Care Medicine* found Honokiol is effective against sepsis, a condition caused by the body's overreaction to injury or infection. In the study, Honokiol reduced reactive oxygen, in the form of nitric oxide, and controlled a number of proteins associated with inflammation to treat life threatening sepsis.

A 2008 study in the journal *Acta Pharmacologica Sinica* demonstrates how Honokiol controls inflammation on the molecular level. By inhibiting proteins associated with the inflammatory enzymes PI3K/Akt, Honokiol provides a significant anti-inflammatory effect.

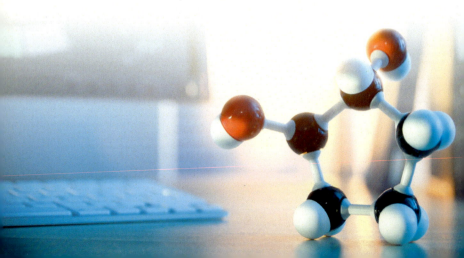

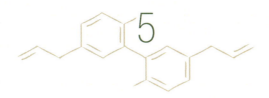

Neural Protection

Honokiol's powerful anti-inflammatory effects extend to the brain. 2012 research published in the *Journal of Neuroinflammation* showed that Honokiol fights inflammation in the brain by inhibiting overactive microglia. Microglia normally defend the brain against infection.

Addressing inflammation is particularly important when treating neurodegenerative conditions such as Alzheimer's disease or dementia. And because Honokiol can cross the blood-brain barrier, it has been shown to be effective against neurological conditions.

Alzheimer's disease deposits thick plaques of amyloid beta protein in the brain. While it's not entirely clear whether this is a cause or an effect of the disease, there's no doubt that these plaques pose a danger to brain health. One 2005 study, published in the journal *Neuroscience Letters*, found that Honokiol's ability to modulate GABA receptors—which we'll discuss more in the next chapter—also helps protect from amyloid beta protein.

In research published in 2000 in the *American Journal of Chinese Medicine*, Honokiol stimulated the neurotransmitter acetylcholine. This is particularly significant because Alzheimer's patients have lower acetylcholine levels.

Research has also confirmed Honokiol's neuro-protective effects against stoke. In one 2012 study in the *Journal of Natural Medicine*, researchers found that Honokiol controlled the glucose intolerance associated with stroke. By reducing glucose intolerance in neurons, Honokiol could potentially prevent cell death; however, Honokiol seems to provide a more comprehensive protection from stroke damage. In a 2007 study in *Basic Clinical Pharmacology and Toxicology*, Honokiol reduced stroke damage by reducing inflammation and oxidation. Still another 2006 study in the *European Journal of Pharmacology* highlighted the overall neuro-protective effects of Honokiol's anti-oxidative effects.

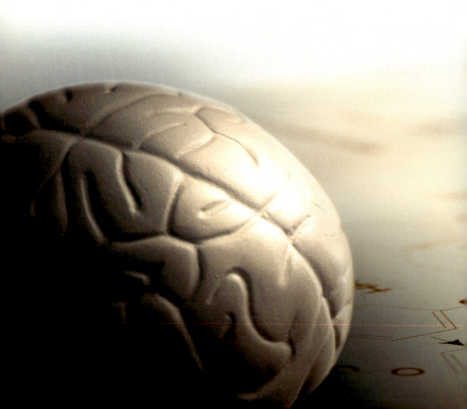

Healthy Mood Support

Because chronic inflammation in the brain is linked to anxiety and depression, it makes sense that Honokiol would address these issues. But it does much more, serving as a gentle yet effective calming agent shown to treat anxiety, depression and occasional insomnia. It works by influencing the activity of certain neurotransmitters in the brain, mainly Gamma-Aminobutyric Acid (GABA), safely and without causing dependency or mental fog.

Historically, one of the most ancient uses of Magnolia bark was to provide a natural, gentle relaxation effect. A variety of studies have indeed confirmed that Honokiol is very useful against both anxiety and depression and does not create dependency or cause side effects.

As noted, Honokiol modulates the neurotransmitter GABA, which helps control electrical activity in the brain and promote a natural relaxation effect. Interestingly, scientists are now finding that modulation of GABA pathways also relates in some ways to cancer prevention and treatment.

Other research has confirmed that Honokiol is equally powerful against depression. The botanical reduced depression symptoms in animals and had a positive impact on neurochemistry.

There has long been an association between anxiety, depression and sleep disorders, so it's not a surprise that Honokiol also benefits sleep. A 2012 study in the *British Journal of Pharmacology* found that small doses of Honokiol extend non-rapid eye movement (REM) sleep by activating neurons at the GABA receptor sites.

Honokiol's ability to influence GABA mechanisms for relaxation has been compared to the anti-anxiety actions of a specific class of pharmaceutical drugs called benzodiazepines. However, these pharmaceuticals (common ones being Valium and Xanax) come with a list of side effects and can be dangerously habit-forming. Honokiol on the other hand, exerts sedative actions that help to relax and calm, without causing dependency, brain fog or toxic effects as prescription drugs often do. A 1999 study in the *Journal of Pharmacy and Pharmacology* showed that Honokiol reduced anxiety comparable to Diazepam (Valium) but did not cause Diazepam-like side effects.

Unfortunately, anxiety and depression are known to worsen other medical conditions, and vice versa — a real catch-22. For example, patients who face a cancer diagnosis must find ways to mitigate their stress or risk a worsened prognosis. Honokiol's ability to calm anxiety could help many patients overcome the stress associated with a serious illness, while its additional benefits help boost health in a number of other areas as well.

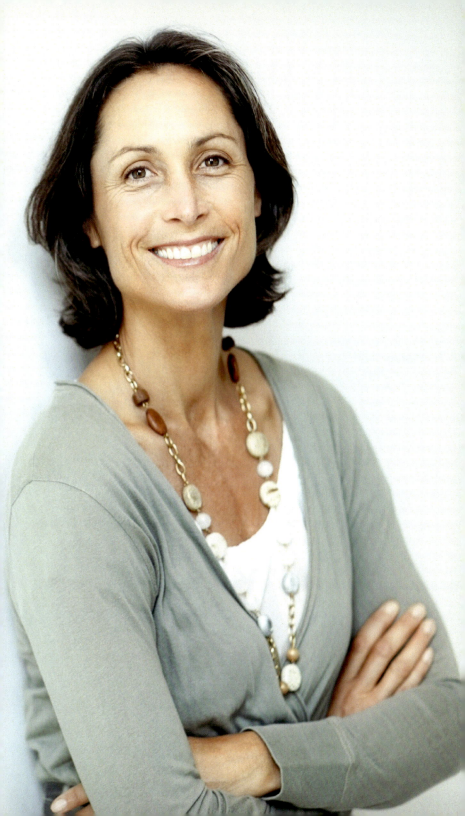

Cardiovascular, Metabolic, Immune Health and more…

While showing powerful activity against cancer, inflammation and anxiety would be enough to earn any treatment high marks, Honokiol has also proven to benefit a number of other conditions. Magnolia bark has a long history in Chinese medicine, dating back nearly 2,000 years to treat gastrointestinal distress, anxiety, respiratory illness and many other issues. On the other side of the East China Sea, Honokiol has been used by traditional Japanese practitioners for its antithrombotic, antibacterial, antidepressant and other effects.

Today, modern research confirms what traditional practitioners have known for millennia—Honokiol offers a wide range of therapeutic benefits beyond cancer alone. It fights cardiovascular disease, balances blood glucose and metabolism, combats infection and more.

Fights Cardiovascular Disease

As noted, oxidative stress has been implicated in many diseases, including heart disease. Oxidation is partially responsible for the arterial plaque accumulation that blocks blood vessels, so we can see where Honokiol's ability to control inflammation and oxidative stress can greatly benefit heart health.

In particular, oxidized LDL cholesterol, the "bad" cholesterol we are so concerned about, creates an inflammatory chain reaction that leads to plaque creation. A number of studies have demonstrated that Honokiol controls LDL oxidation, mitigating these negative effects.

In addition, Honokiol also exhibits characteristics found in pharmaceutical blood thinners. By controlling platelets, the blood components responsible for clotting, Honokiol can help prevent the arterial blockages that lead to cardiovascular disease.

Hypertension, or high blood pressure, is also a risk factor for heart disease. Again, Honokiol can help. A study published in 2010 in the *Biological Pharmaceutical Bulletin* showed that Honokiol can significantly reduce blood pressure.

Treats Kidney Disease

The buildup of fibrous tissue in kidney, or renal fibrosis, is a major component of kidney disease and can impair the ability of kidneys to function. This degenerative condition often leads to eventual kidney failure. A 2011 study in the *British Journal of Pharmacology* showed that Honokiol acts against a variety of proteins known to cause renal fibrosis.

Anti-microbial Actions

The fight against pathogens, particularly bacteria and viruses, is ongoing. Because they mutate so rapidly, these invaders can be difficult to treat. Flu viruses change every season and bacteria develop resistance to frontline antibiotics. Eastern medicine has long recognized Honokiol's ability to fight pathogens, and new research is substantiating this important application.

Viruses can be particularly troublesome. They inject genetic material into cells, hijacking the cellular replication processes in order to make more viruses. A study published in the journal *Liver International* showed that Honokiol short-circuits this process, preventing the Hepatitis C (Hep C) virus from infecting cells. By locking Hep C outside the cell, Honokiol prevents it from completing its life cycle.

Honokiol has shown similar potent antibacterial action, particularly against the bacteria associated with periodontal disease, such as *Porphyromonas gingivalis, Prevotella intermedia, Micrococcus luteus, Bacillus subtilis* and others.

Stimulates Glucose Metabolism

Metabolic syndrome and its sinister offspring, type 2 diabetes, starts when cells have trouble taking in blood sugar, or glucose. When glucose rises, the pancreas pumps out more insulin to tell cells to take in more glucose. As the cycle proceeds, cells become more insulin-resistant, the pancreas works harder and harder, and too much glucose remains outside cells, damaging blood vessels and tissues throughout the body.

Research published in 2012 in the journal *Biofactors* demonstrates that Honokiol can break this cycle by helping cells to absorb more glucose. In addition, Honokiol optimizes insulin signaling, the messages that tell cells to take in sugar in the first place. This combined effect has a great impact on insulin signaling and could be very helpful in treating both type 2 diabetes and metabolic syndrome.

Bio-Activity

One of the major concerns in medical care is targeting the right treatments to the right areas of the body. Sometimes a compound may have promising attributes in a test tube but, when it is used in a living organism, its molecules are too large to work as was hoped. This is critically important and one of the reasons Honokiol is so effective against so many conditions.

Honokiol exhibits extreme bio-activity. In other words, its molecules are small enough to easily enter the blood stream and quickly reach targeted areas, such as tumors, arterial blockages, fibrous kidneys and even the brain. Honokiol travels throughout the circulation for maximum therapeutic benefit.

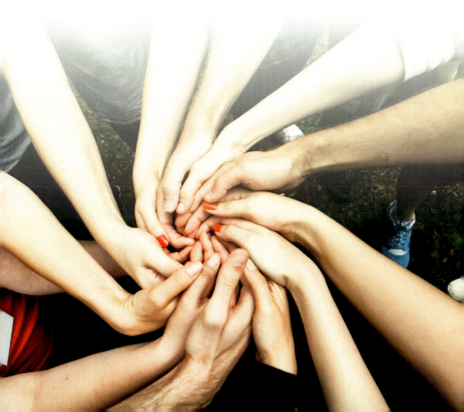

The Future of Honokiol

You may have known about Honokiol before reading this guide. Or, this might have been the first time you ever heard of this fascinating ingredient. Either way, you will be hearing much more about this remarkable botanical therapy as research continues to uncover and substantiate its numerous critical benefits.

The wide range of published data cited here is only the tip of the iceberg. Hundreds of studies have shown Honokiol's effectiveness against many conditions. More research is currently being conducted, and still more studies are being planned. Needless to say, future editions of this guide will be updated to reflect these new findings.

What's most important is how this knowledge is being translated into patient care. For the medical profession, a treatment that works against cancer, heart disease, mood disorders, inflammation and oxidation—without side effects—may have seemed too good to be true. But as published research and clinical reports continue to substantiate Honokiol's beneficial effects, more practitioners are integrating this important botanical therapy into their clinical protocols. From medical professionals to savvy health-seekers, Honokiol is steadily gaining a well-earned

Chapter 8: The Future of Honokiol

reputation, offering new hope and a powerful advantage in achieving optimal long term wellness and vitality. Stay tuned for further advancements along this exciting, cutting-edge of modern botanical medicine.

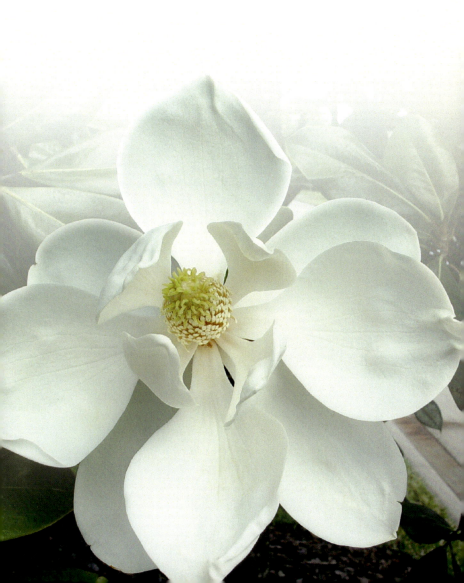

Appendix i

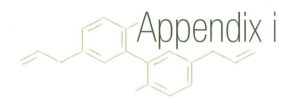

How to Use Honokiol

Honokiol Dosages	
Active Cancer	Build up to 1 gram, 3 times per day starting with 250 mg, 3 times per day. Can be increased as directed by healthcare provider
Prevention and Post Therapy	1 gram per day
Anti-inflammatory and Circulation Support	250 mg, 2 times per day to 500 mg, 2 times per day
Periodontal Disease	500 mg, 2 times per day until condition improves; then 250 mg, 2 times per day
Antioxidant	250 mg, 2 times per day
Anxiety	250 mg, 2 times per day
Sleep	250 mg before bed

Best taken with food. Increase dose gradually by one to two capsules per day.

Frequently Asked Questions

What makes Honokiol different than magnolia bark?

Purified Honokiol, the active ingredient in magnolia bark extract, is much more powerful than the whole plant. When Honokiol is used in combination with other botanicals and nutrients which have similar or complementary communication functions, the effects of each component are enhanced beyond the effects of the individual components.

Should Honokiol be taken on an empty stomach or with food?

Honokiol can be taken with or without food but, due to the potential for stomach upset at higher doses, it is best taken with food.

Can you build up a resistance to Honokiol?

This has not been seen in the literature.

Are there any contraindication or cautions for Honokiol?

Honokiol helps to relax. If serious drowsiness occurs, do not drive or operate machinery until you feel alert. This effect may be increased by alcohol, sleeping aids or sedatives.

In very rare cases, itchiness or rash may occur. If this happens, discontinue use.

If you are nursing, pregnant or considering pregnancy, you should consult your healthcare practitioner prior to using this product.

Rare mild digestive discomfort at high doses can be alleviated with appropriate digestive support.

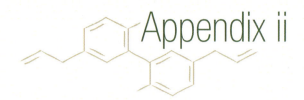

Appendix ii

References & Research

Alexeev M, Grosenbaugh DK, Mott DD, Fisher JL. The natural products magnolol and honokiol are positive allosteric modulators of both synaptic and extra-synaptic GABA(A) receptors.Neuropharmacology. 2012 Jun;62(8):2507-14. Epub 2012 Mar 12.

Angelini A, Di Ilio C, Castellani ML, Conti P, Cuccurullo F. Modulation of multidrug resistance p-glycoprotein activity by flavonoids and honokiol in human doxorubicin-resistant sarcoma cells (MES-SA/DX-5): implications for natural sedatives as chemosensitizing agents in cancer therapy. J Biol Regul Homeost Agents. 2010 Apr-Jun;24(2):197-205.

Arora S, Bhardwaj A, Srivastava SK, Singh S, McClellan S, Wang B, Singh AP. Honokiol arrests cell cycle, induces apoptosis, and potentiates the cytotoxic effect of gemcitabine in human pancreatic cancer cells. PLoS ONE. 2011 6(6): e21573. doi:10.1371/journal.pone.0021573.

Chang B, Lee Y, Ku Y, Bae K, Chung C. Antimicrobial activity of magnolol and honokiol against periodontopathic microorganisms. Planta Med. 1998 May; 64(4):367-9.

Chen C M, Liu S H, Lin-Shiau SY. Honokiol, a neuroprotectant against mouse cerebral ischemia, mediated by preserving Na+, K+-ATPase activity and mitochondrial functions. Basic Clin Pharmacol Toxicol. 2007 Aug;101(2);108-16.

Chen XR, Lu R, Dan HX, Liao G, Zhou M, Li XY, Ji N. Honokiol: a promising small molecular weight natural agent for the growth inhibition of oral squamous cell carcinoma cells. Int J Oral Sci. 2011 Jan;3(1):34-42. doi: 10.4248/IJOS11014.

Cheng N, Xia T, Han Y, He QJ, Zhao R, Ma JR. Synergistic antitumor effects of liposomal honokiol combined with cisplatin in colon cancer models. Oncol Lett. 2011 Sep 1;2(5):957-962. Epub 2011 Jul 5.

Chiang CK, Sheu ML, Lin YW, Wu CT, Yang CC, Chen MW, Hung KY, Wu KD, Liu SH. Honokiol ameliorates renal fibrosis by inhibiting extracellular matrix and pro-inflammatory factors in vivo and in vitro. Br J Pharmacol. 2011 Jun;163(3):586-97. doi: 10.1111/j.1476-5381.2011.01242.x.

Chilampalli S, Zhang X, Fahmy H, Kaushik RS, Zeman D, Hildreth MB, Dwivedi C. Chemopreventive effects of honokiol on UVB-induced skin cancer development. Anti-cancer Res. 2010 Mar;30(3):777-83.

Choi SS, Cha BY, Lee YS, Yonezawa T, Teruya T, Nagai K, Woo JT. Honokiol and magnolol stimulate glucose uptake by activating PI3K-dependent Akt in L6 myotubes. Biofactors. 2012 Sep;38(5):372-7. doi: 10.1002/biof.1029. Epub 2012 Jun 7.

Dikalov S, Losik T, Arbiser JL. Honokiol is a potent scavenger of superoxide and peroxyl radicals. Biochem Pharmacol. 2008 Sep 1;76(5):589-96. Epub 2008 Jul 2.

Fried LE, Arbiser JL. Honokiol, a multifunctional antiangiogenic and antitumor agent. Antioxid Redox Signal. 2009 May;11(5):1139-48. doi: 10.1089/ARS.2009.2440.

Guillermo RF, Chilampalli C, Zhang Z, Zeman D, Fahmy H, Dwivedi C. Time and dose-response effects of honokiol on UVB-induced skin cancer development. Drug Discov Ther. 2012 Jun;6(3):140-6.

Harada S, Kishimoto M, Kobayashi M, Nakamoto K, Fujita-Hamabe W, Chen HH, Chan MH, Tokuyama S. Honokiol suppresses the development of post-ischemic glucose intolerance and neuronal damage in mice. J Nat Med. 2012 Oct;66(4):591-9. doi: 10.1007/s11418-011-0623-x. Epub 2012 Jan 20.

He Z, Subramaniam D, Ramalingam S, Dhar A, Postier RG, Umar S, Zhang Y, Anant S. Honokiol radiosensitizes colorectal cancer cells: enhanced activity in cells with mismatch repair defects. Am J Physiol Gastrointest Liver Physiol. 2011 Nov;301(5):G929-37. doi: 10.1152/ajpgi.00159.2011. Epub 2011 Aug 11.

Hou, Y. C., Chao, P. D., & Chen, S. Y. Honokiol and magnolol increased hippocampal acetylcholine release in freely-moving rats. Am J Chin Med . 2000;28(3-4):379–384.

Ishikawa C, Arbiser JL, Mori N. Honokiol induces cell cycle arrest and apoptosis via inhibition of survival signals in adult T-cell leukemia. Biochim Biophys Acta. 2012 Jul;1820(7):879-87.

Kaushik DK, Mukhopadhyay R, Kumawat KL, Gupta M, Basu A. Therapeutic targeting of Krüppel-like factor 4 abrogates microglial activation. J Neuroinflammation. 2012 Mar 19;9:57. doi: 10.1186/1742-2094-9-57.

Kaushik G, Ramalingam S, Subramanium D, Rangarajan P, Protti P, Rammamoorthy P, Anant S, Mammen JM. Honokiol induces cytotoxic and cytostatic effects in malignant melanoma cancer cells. Am J Surg. 2012 Dec;204(6):868-73.

Kim BH, Cho JY. Anti-inflammatory effect of honokiol is mediated by PI3K, Akt pathway suppression. Acta Pharmacol Sin. 2008 Jan;29(1):113-22.

Kuribara H, Stavinoha WB, Maruyama Y. Honokiol, a putative anxiolytic agent extracted from magnolia bark, has no diazepam-like side-effects in mice. J Pharm Pharmacol. 1999 Jan;51(1):97-103.

Lan KH, Wang YW, Lee WP, Lan KL, Tseng SH, Hung LR, Yen SH, Lin HC, Lee SD. Multiple effects of honokiol on the life cycle of hepatitis C virus. Liver Int. 2012 Jul;32(6):989-97. doi: 10.1111/j.1478-3231.2011.02621.x Epub 2011 Aug 11.

Lee J, Jung E, Park J, Jung K, Lee S, Hong S, Park J, Park E, Kim J, Park S, Park D. Anti-inflammatory effects of magnolol and honokiol are mediated through inhibition of the downstream pathway of MEKK-1 in NF-kappaB activation signaling. Planta Med. 2005 Apr;71(4):338-43.

Lee YJ, Lee YM, Lee CK, Jung JK, Han SB, Hong JT. Therapeutic applications of compounds in the Magnolia family. Pharmacol Ther. 2011 May;130(2):157-76. Epub 2011 Jan 26.

Lin YR, Chen HH, Ko CH, Chan MH. Neuroprotective activity of honokiol and magnolol in cerebellar granule cell damage. Eur J Pharmacol. 2006 May 10;537(1-3):64-9. Epub 2006 Mar 24.

Liou KT, Shen YC, Chen CF, Tsao CM, Tsai SK. The anti-inflammatory effect of honokiol on neutrophils: mechanisms in the inhibition of reactive oxygen species production. Eur J Pharmacol. 2003 Aug 15;475(1-3):19-27.

Liu B, Hattori N, Zhang NY, Wu B, Yang L, Kitagawa K, Xiong ZM, Irie T, Inagaki C. Anxiolytic agent, dihydrohonokiol-B, recovers amyloid beta protein-induced neurotoxicity in cultured rat hippocampal neurons. Neurosci Lett. 2005 Aug 12-19;384(1-2):44-7.

Liu SH, Wang KB, Lan KH, Lee WJ, Pan HC, Wu SM, Peng YC, Chen YC, Shen CC, Cheng HC, Liao KK, Sheu ML. Calpain/SHP-1 interaction by honokiol dampening peritoneal dissemination of gastric cancer in nu/nu mice. PLoS One. 2012;7(8):e43711.

Nagalingam A, Arbiser JL, Bonner MY, Saxena NK, Sharma D. Honokiol activates AMP-activated protein kinase in breast cancer cells via an LKB1-dependent pathway and inhibits breast carcinogenesis. Breast Cancer Res. 2012 Feb 21;14(1):R35.

Park J, Lee J, Jung E, Park Y, Kim K, Park B, Jung K, Park E, Kim J, Park D. In vitro antibacterial and anti-inflammatory effects of honokiol and magnolol against Propionibacterium sp. Eur J Pharmacol. 2004 Aug 2;496(1-3):189-95.

Ponnurangam S, Mammen JM, Ramalingam S, He Z, Zhang Y, Umar S, Subramaniam D, Anant S. Honokiol in combination with radiation targets notch signaling to inhibit colon cancer stem cells. Mol Cancer Ther. 2012 Apr;11(4):963-72. doi: 10.1158/1535-7163.MCT-11-0999. Epub 2012 Feb 8.

Qu WM, Yue XF, Sun Y, Fan K, Chen CR, Hou YP, Urade Y, Huang ZL. Honokiol promotes non-rapid eye movement sleep via the benzodiazepine site of the GABA(A) receptor in mice.

Br J Pharmacol. 2012 Oct;167(3):587-98. doi: 10.1111/j.1476-5381.2012.02010.

Schäfer-Korting M, Korting HC, Lukacs A, Heykants J, Behrendt H. Levels of itraconazole in skin blister fluid after a single oral dose and during repetitive administration. J Am Acad Dermatol. 1990 Feb;22(2 Pt 1):211-5.

Singh T, Prasad R, Katiyar SK. Inhibition of class 1 histone deacetylases in non-small cell lung cancer by honokiol leads to suppression of cancer cell growth and induction of cell death in vitro and in vivo. Epigenetics. 2013 Jan1;8(1):54-65.

Steinmann P, Walters DK, Arlt MJ, Banke IJ, Ziegler U, Langsam B, Arbiser J, Muff R, Born W, Fuchs B. Antimetastatic activity of honokiol in osteosarcoma. Cancer. 2012 Apr 15;118(8): 2117-27.

Tian W, Deng Y, Li L, He H, Sun J, Xu D. Honokiol synergizes chemotherapy drugs in multidrug resistant breast cancer cells via enhanced apoptosis and additional programmed necrotic death. Int J Oncol. 2013 Feb;42(2):721-32.

Wang X, Duan X, Yang G, Zhang X, Deng L, Zheng H, Deng C, Wen J, Wang N, Peng C, Zhao X, Wei Y, Chen L. Honokiol crosses BBB and BCSFB, and inhibits brain tumor growth in rat 9L intracerebral gliosarcoma model and human U251 xenograft glioma model. PLoS One. 2011 Apr 29;6(4):e18490. doi: 10.1371/journal.pone.0018490.

Want Y, Yang Z, Zhao Z. Honokiol induces parapoptosis and apoptosis and exhibits schedule-dependent synergy in combination with imatinib in human leukemia cells. Toxicol Mech Methods. 2010 Jun;20(5):234-41.

Weng TI, Wu HY, Kuo CW, Liu SH. Honokiol rescues sepsis-associated acute lung injury and lethality via the inhibition of oxidative stress and inflammation. Intensive Care Med. 2011 Mar;37(3):533-41. Epub 2011 Jan 29.

Xu HL, Tang W, Du GH, Kokudo N. Targeting apoptosis pathways in cancer with magnolol and honokiol, bioactive constituents of the bark of Magnolia officinalis. Drug Discov Ther. 2011 Oct;5(5):202-10.

Xu Q, Yi LT, Pan Y, Wang X, Li YC, Li JM, Wang CP, Kong LD. Antidepressant-like effects of the mixture of honokiol and magnolol from the barks of Magnolia officinalis in stressed rodents.

Prog Neuropsychopharmacol Biol Psychiatry. 2008 Apr 1;32(3):715-25. Epub 2007 Nov 28.

Zhang GS, Wang RJ, Zhang HN, Zhang GP, Luo MS, Luo JD. Effects of chronic treatment with honokiol in spontaneously hypertensive rats. Bio Pharm Bull. 2010;33(3):427-31.

Zhao C, Liu ZQ. Comparison of antioxidant abilities of magnolol and honokiol to scavenge radicals and to protect DNA. Biochimie. 2011 Oct;93(10):1755-60. Epub 2011 Jun 23.

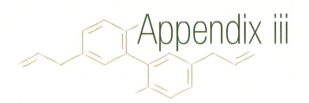

Appendix iii

Index

A

Acetylcholine 16
Alzheimer's Disease 15, 16
Anti-anxiety ii, 17, 18, 20
Antibacterial ii, 20, 22
Antibiotics 21
Antidepressant ii, 17, 18, 20
Anti-inflammatory ii, 1, 14, 15
Anti-metastasis ii, 2, 3, 8
Antioxidant ii, 1, 13
Anti-tumor ii, 2, 3, 8, 23
Anxiety ii, 17, 18, 20
Apoptosis 3, 4, 6, 7, 8
Arterial Plaque 14, 20, 21

B

Bacteria 2, 21, 22
Blood-Brain Barrier 2, 15
Blood Pressure 21
Bone Cancer 3, 4
Brain Tumor 2, 3
Breast Cancer 3, 11

C

Cardiovascular Disease ii, 14, 20, 21
Cell Cycle 6, 7, 8
Cell Signaling 3, 7
Chemotherapy ii, 1, 4, 10, 11, 12
Chemotherapy Resistance 1
Circulation 2, 23
Cisplatin 12
Colon Cancer 3, 12

D

Dementia 15
Depression 17, 18
DNA 2, 6, 13
Doxorubicin 12

F

Free Radical 1, 13

G

GABA 15, 17, 18
Gastric Cancer 3
Gemcitabine 6, 12
Gliosarcoma 2
Glucose ii, 16, 20, 22

H

Heart Disease 13, 14, 20, 21, 24
Hepatitis C 22
Hypertension 21

I

Imatinib 12
Immunity ii, 2, 13, 14, 20
Infection 2, 14, 15, 20
Inflammation 1, 5, 8, 13, 14, 15, 16, 17, 20, 24
Insomnia 17
Insulin 22
Integrative Oncology i

K

Kidney Disease 21

L

LDL Cholesterol 21
Leukemia 3, 7, 12
Lung Cancer 3, 7

M

Magnolia i, 17, 20
Melanoma 3, 7
Metabolic Syndrome 22
Metabolism 20, 22
Metastasis ii, 2, 3, 8
Microglia 15
Modified Citrus Pectin 12

N

NF-kB 8
Nitric Oxide 14

O

Oral Cancer 3
Oxidation 1, 2, 5, 8, 13, 14, 16, 20, 21, 24

P

P53 8
Pancreas 22
Periodontal Disease 22
Platelets 21
Proliferation 3, 6, 7, 8, 12
Prostate Cancer 3, 11, 12

R

Radiation ii, 1, 4, 11, 12
Reactive Oxygen 13, 14
Renal Fibrosis 21

S

Sepsis 14
Skin Cancer 3
Stroke 14, 16
Synergy 8, 10

T

Traditional Chinese Medicine i, 20
Treatment Resistance 1, 10, 11, 21, 27
Type 2 Diabetes 22

V

Viruses 21
Vitamin E 13